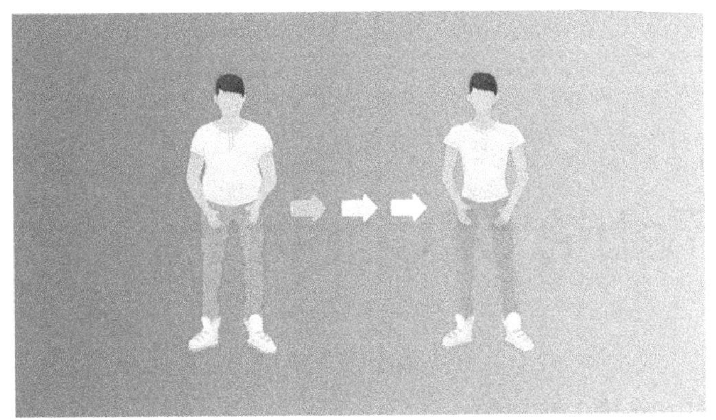

Lose Weight,

Feel Great -

get your weight

under control

Table of Contents

About the author

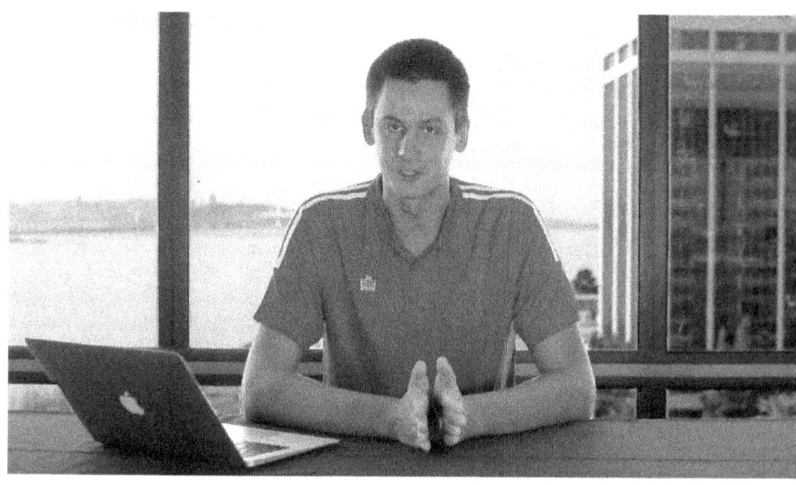

Vasily is a Product Manager living and working in San Francisco Bay Area. He is currently leading Tesla Digital Order Management team. Before joining Tesla, for three years Vasily led Driver Growth and Driver Experience products at Uber. Prior to that, Vasily led consumer product at Reputation.com and worked for number of late

stage VC funded Silicon Valley startups:
SuccessFactors, BitTorrent and others

In his career, Vasily is primarily focusing on solving large complex problems and profitable growth. His top interests are product experimentation, understanding customer needs, managing a product for maximum impact, and what defines and makes product successful. To satisfy these interests, Vasily is advising and investing in startups, teaching online and helping startup employees navigate complex topics such as employee equity.

Vasily has MBA from Stanford Graduate School of Business and holds Master degrees in Physics from Moscow Institute of Physics and Technology and Economics from New Economic School. Vasily loves large numbers, is a big fan of operations and operational excellence. Vasily is a proponent of

living healthy, he is a former competitive swimmer

and Champion of Moscow Region in Swimming

Introduction

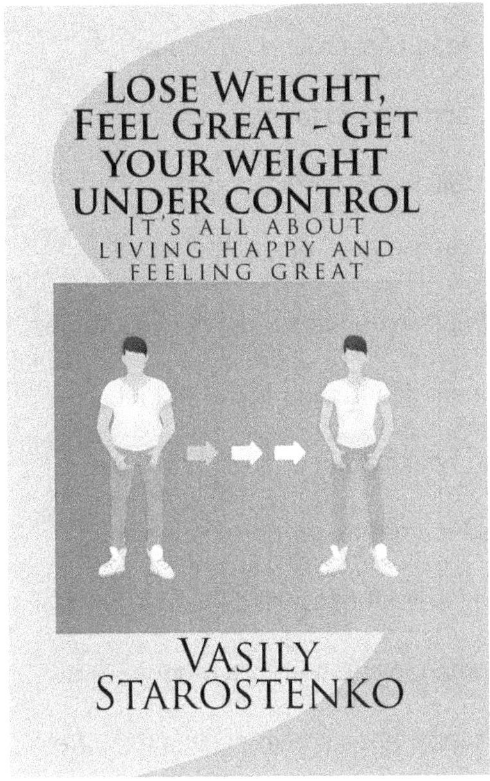

Welcome to my first book, the book about weight

management, a topic I'm deeply passionate about.

My name is Vasily and I work as a Product Manager in Silicon Valley: currently leading customer acquisition for Tesla, previously did Driver Growth for Uber, lead consumer products at Reputation.com, and worked for number of late stage VC funded Silicon Valley startups: SuccessFactors, BitTorrent and others.

In this book I'm truly excited to share with you some of the most fascinating learnings about weight management and health that I acquired over the last five years as I started to be more conscious about weight and health. I converted these learnings to become tools to be more productive at work in general happy in life so I'm excited to share those learnings with you and hear your feedback.

To start this book I would like to share with you a statement that Russian people often make. They say "You know it is a lot better to be both wealthy

and healthy than to be poor and sick". And honestly

given that I have a critical mind and most of the

statements I hear, I usually try to argue with this

one there is no way I could argue with this one. Let

us get both healthy and wealthy.

Right, it is really good to be wealthy and healthy

and the even more important thing about health is

you cannot get it back immediately once you've lost

it. That's how it is profoundly different from wealth

and weight to me is one major attribute of health

staying in a healthy weight allows you to feel great

and allows you to be more healthy that's why this

course is about weight management.

As we talk about weight management we will

obviously mostly focus on weight loss because for

many people the problem is an excess weight and losing weight.

However, I hope that most of the learnings and most of the principles we're going to discuss most of the definitions will be applicable to other kinds of weight management. For instance, these other kinds of weight management can be: muscle gain, it can be a simple maintenance of weight level you have, or it may be some kind of toning getting your stomach flatter and your abs show up better etc.

In this book we will together discover several pretty exciting things. Let us get started

What this book is about

There are several key topics I want to cover in this book.

First, I want to discuss the best thing about weight management.

Second, I want to talk to you about the worst thing about weight management.

Third, I want to go and talk about exercise and in particular exercise as not a weight management tool.

Today mainly fitness clubs are promoting exercise , and people are enrolling in fitness classes in the beginning of the year only to disenroll later and break expectations. So I really want to communicate this point to you that they do not believe that exercise is a good weight management tool. it is a great health tool it is a great wellness tool but they do not think it is a great weight management tool.

Fourth, I want to talk to you about my personal experience managing weight and in particular losing more than 50 pounds each time of the course of last 50 years. Most recently it is basically happening right now I'm moving into the maintenance mode and I want to talk to you about how different those two experiences were and what they learned in the process.

And then ultimately I want to talk to you about fasting and calorie restrictions. And probably a little bit about the food diets and also describe what worked for me and what did not work for me. And I think this is going to be in the most exciting part of this book, so let us start.

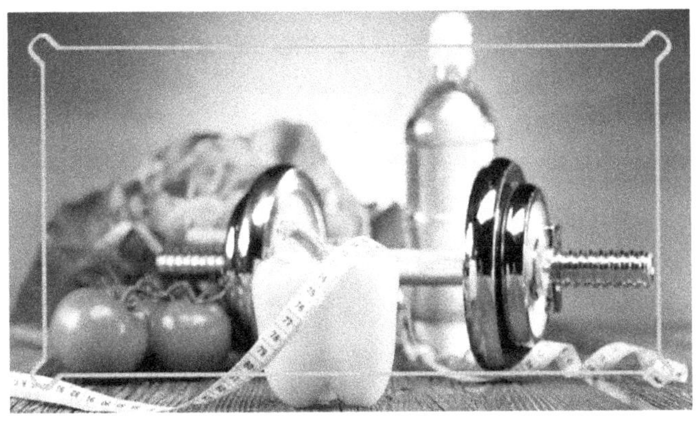

The best thing about weight management

Now let us talk about the best thing about weight management. The best thing about weight management is that **there is a guaranteed way to succeed**. For everyone. Anyone can do it and if you are doing the right thing you can be confident that ultimately you will get what you want there is

no probabilities. There is no chance of not

succeeding.

Guaranteed Way to Succeed

it is all about sticking to the rules figuring out what works for you and just going the whole way. it is important to emphasize the long term and keep totally clear: it is a journey, you cannot get it all done in a day or two. You can probably not get it done in a week or in a month.

Get ready for the long journey as you generally should be thinking about life and your career anyway so I'm assuming this kind of thinking is not new for most of us. So think about weight management as another long term journey you need to take upon. You need to keep improving as you take on this journey, then you will be successful: there is no chance you are not going to succeed.

This is by far the best thing about weight management. And for example can be compared with some other things such as learning a new skill learning a new subject. You can try really hard but in many cases you are just not capable of doing that even if you apply high effort over a long period of time. So in this case your effort can potentially be wasted or even if not wasted that it does not bring you as much satisfaction as you wanted. Or alternative example for instance in health is some of the diseases are not curable and you can spend as much money as you want and you can spend as much time as you want on trying to cure it and it is not going to work. That is luckily not the case with weight management.

Weight management to me is not rocket science it is a **<u>pure deterministic effort and discipline</u>** and just following certain rules and figuring out what works for you. But also it is a good way for you to learn that you are disciplined enough and you can manage certain things that we did not previously believe you can or should even manage.

So let us get there and also we start talking about what weight management is, once again the best thing about weight management is the fact that it is deterministic.

I really want to make several statements that for some people it is going to be more difficult than for other people. Because there could be complications when it is not just about reducing the amount of fat in your body through creating an energy deficit.

The Law of Conservation of Energy

And talking about fat, fat is just a form of stored energy and we are talking about the law of conservation of energy which is the universal physical law. Anybody in the universe obeys this law including your human body. There is nothing that can disobey the law of energy conservation. So in the human body the energy conservation works by storing fat when you take more energy in than you can spend.

If you eat too much, the fat gets stored. If you do not eat too much you do not gain any fat. If you do not eat enough then your body will start burning stored fat and potentially muscle tissue and some other substances you can find in the body such as bacteria, viruses, and other things.

So let us talk about what kind of complications

there can be when weight management may be a

little bit more difficult than I'm trying to present your

now.

Sometimes for instance your body may be polluted

with heavy metals or some other bad substances.

And in those cases fat can be used as a tool to

store those bad substances to not expose your vital

organs to them and keep you healthy. In this case

your body will be trying to fight really hard when

you try to reduce fat because the substances in fact

will be damaging to your body. Ideally, you will

need to find a way to clean up your body before

trying to reduce the amount of fat. Otherwise when

these bad substances get into your blood you will

have to go through potentially lengthy periods of

headache and feeling not great.

The other complications may include bacterial microflora as well as some parasitic infections which can go as far as potentially directly influence your brain and just force you crave certain kinds of foods in a way you cannot control or avoid. So in those cases again it still is deterministic you can make through this if you keep going and do whatever is right to enjoy success at the end of the journey.

But the journey is going to be more difficult in this case and those complications may present really substantial hurdles to you, so be ready. And it will require a lot of discipline and a lot of self-motivation to just keep doing what you are doing. To not break the rule and to not get back into the habits that were not good for your weight early on.

So given these things let us talk about it in a little bit more detail why is weight management and weight loss a deterministic process and everyone is guaranteed to succeed. As I mentioned previously, there is a law of conservation of energy and this law is universal enough so that no one can break this law. And if it is convincing enough then you can just take it from there. If it is not convincing enough and you do not believe in laws of physics, and you need more clear demonstration of this fact working, then I'm going to give you an example.

Probably not the most exciting example, but it is often cited in the literature. Some people say for instance that they are not prone to weight loss and actually prone to weight gain. They say "My DNA and my genetics are such that I just gain weight easily and it is impossible to lose it after that" and those people usually just use it as an excuse.

Excuse that I do not feel good with this weight but

unfortunately there is nothing I can do about it is

just my destiny and I have to live with it.

So there is an example to prove these people

wrong and this example is from the military times in

concentration camps. You see the pictures and all

the people look pretty horrific, they look there is no

fat on them they look pretty thin and exhausted.

You can be confident that many many different

people made it in the concentration camp. Some of

them were fat, some of them were obese, some

were normal weight.

But in the end they all end up looking exactly

identical, so you can see that a lot of work, bad

conditions. and also not enough food will eventually

turn you into something like what you see on those

pictures. Guaranteed. So again body transformation when exposed to continuous energy deficit it is a pretty deterministic straightforward process which anyone can use to their benefit. And I would love you to use it to your benefit.

So now let us talk about energy conservation. There is IN and OUT in energy equation, and IN is basically your food intake. When you eat food your body converts this food into energy during digestion and further processing in intestines. And different kinds of food can be converted into different amounts of energy so body uses this energy for different purposes. Body more easily stores some of kinds of energy and more easily uses some other kinds of energy for work. This is regulated by hormones and often measured through glycemic and insulinemic indices. You can read about it in the literature and I'm not going to go deep into this topic here.

There is so much literature on the subject which foods you should eat, when, and which you should not and when that I assume you will find good sources.

There is also lots of diets I'm not spending too much time on this in my book simply because one is I'm not a big believer diets and most diabetologists I respect give a similar advice. I really do not think for many people diets are good weight management tool. Because those diets result in extra constraints and limitations that you do not want to handle, not to mention they may create deficit of nutrients your body needs.

Ultimately you are not going to be able to handle sticking to the diet for too long.

So energy IN is the food you eat, energy OUT is

what your body consumes and your body

consumes energy on many different things.

First of all it needs to run itself during the day and

the amount of energy the body spends during the

day simply on its vital process it is called basal

metabolic rate or BMR. There are four important

organs which consume most of energy:

- brain is up to 20%

- heart is also roughly around 20%

- liver

- lungs

Four of those organs together consume roughly

80% of all of your basal metabolic rate. All other

organs including muscles do not really consume

too much. So your body mostly needs energy for those four vital organs.

And then all the energy you spend walking, breathing, and moving during the day. Usually this total amount of energy including BMR + Active is somewhere between two and three thousand (kilo) calories (1 kilocalories is normally called a calorie on food labels).

Daily energy spend is different for different people depending on weight, age, gender but it is roughly again between two and three thousand for normal people. For some people like sportsmen, it could go up to five and six thousand or more. It can be ridiculous large amounts for example Michael Phelps was known to burn 12,000 calories a day - an amount normal person burns in a week.

To put things in perspective for instance one burrito would be a thousand calories. One hamburger could be something like thousand calories so this was pretty shocking for me to learn that actually a very small amount of food can be enough for you to run your body the whole day without tapping into energy stores. Especially if this day is not the most active day for you, and without knowing this if you just keep eating the way your cultural norms suggest it is really easy for you to break the energy balance in a sense that what you get in cannot be spent out.

In this case you will be storing fat as a form of energy in your body. And in this case this fat will be accumulating over time and it will making you feel slower and make you basically feel a less and less great over time. But there is not much you can do about it until you change your eating habits.

This was the best thing about weight management and the best thing about weight management is the fact that anyone can do it. The fact that you are guaranteed to succeed and the fact that this is not a rocket science so anyone can do it.

You are guaranteed to succeed you just need to figure out what works for you. You need to figure out what energy in what energy out you can afford and what energy in and out you need to do and how many pounds we need to get gone.

And then we just need to again plan for a long journey. It is a very important part of this book: it is not about two days magic diet to lose five pounds for a class party or something.

This book is about building sustainable habits, explaining to you which rules work, explaining to you that the long term mindset is the key to success. Not just in life, not just with your health but also with your weight management efforts. And as soon as you understand this and as soon as you internalize this mindset and you are ready to go. Energy IN - energy OUT: the Delta is basically your daily caloric deficit or surplus. Depending on what it is, and then depending on how many pounds you need to get gone (1 pound of fat is roughly 3,500 calories) you can just do your math. You can understand what calorie deficit over the what period of time can take you there.

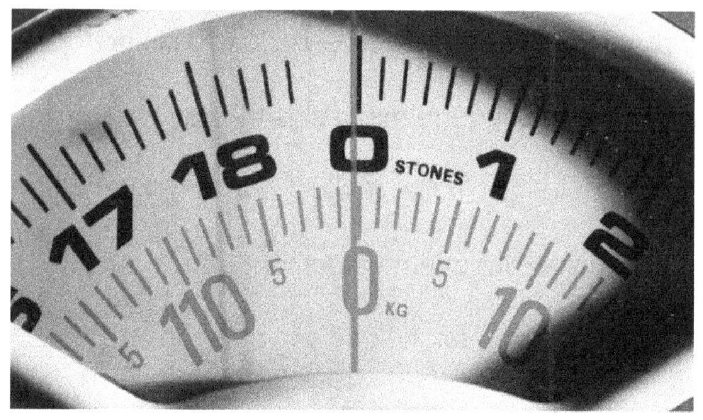

The worst thing about

weight management

Let us talk about the worst thing about weight management. This worst thing about weight management is actually pretty annoying and I was personally annoyed with it for a long, long time. Until I learned to deal with it in some way, whether that's the best way or not. But I'm going to share it

with you and you can judge it and you can share

with me what you think about it.

So what is the worst thing about weight

management?

You Manage What You Measure

First of all in any kind of management it is important that you know what outcome you are aiming at and it is critical that there is some kind of a metric that you are targeting.

My favorite professor in business school used to teach me that you only manage what you measure. And in ideal world you only measure what you manage, as you generally do not want to measure other things. Because otherwise you are just going to end up with lots of numbers which make no sense.

So, in this case what you need to understand first is what we're trying to measure. And obviously if we are talking the weight management, so probably we are trying to measure our weight, right?

Let us say you weigh 200 pounds and you want this number to go down to become 190, and then 180, then 170 etc. So that's the number we are looking to manage and measuring this number needs to make sense. And probably it does, right? Because ultimately this is this is what we are trying to move up or down and this is a single most important metric in this whole exercise. Assuming other critically important metrics such as your overall health, attitude, energy level and others stay the same or improve as well.

However, the challenges start immediately. Your weight depends on a number of factors as your body is composed of distinct and very different components. Those are for instance the muscle mass. the fat mass, and also the amount of water in your body. Water is the dominant part of your body in terms of your total body weight, and generally

amounts to about 60% of your total weight.

But not only water represents such a large fraction

of your total weight, it also fluctuates a lot and

makes it difficult to understand in which direction

your muscle weight and fat weight are changing.

Also, if you exercise for instance you might gain

muscle, which is good for your body. But when you

step on the scale you may see that the weight is

not going down, and that can be really frustrating.

But in fact this new muscle weight you gained is

good for you.

This muscle makes you stronger, it makes you

actually feel good even if fat is not going away. And

it also quietly burns calories over the course of the

day so it increases your metabolic rate and it

makes you more of a burning machine. In terms of

numbers, a pound of muscle burns roughly 10 extra calories per day, which translates into an extra pound of weight loss during the course of the year other things being equal. 10 extra calories over 365 days = 3,650 calories which well compares with amount of energy one pound of body fat contains. So new muscle makes you more efficient at maintaining your health and maintaining your weight.

But other than muscle, there is also water in your body and the water weight creates a big, big problem for your weight management effort, because the water weight varies a lot and is hard to observe or measure. The variation can be in many cases as high as 10 pounds over the course of just several days. You can be doing a really great job counting your calories or maybe exercising or maybe spending more energy. But sometimes the weight just simply does not change, or in the worst case scenario it may actually go up which is completely counterintuitive and can drive you crazy. And this is actually super, super frustrating. You exhibit best of your discipline, limiting your food intake and trying to eat vegetables instead of this great steak and not drinking alcohol, which is insane amount of energy.

You are doing your best, not eating sugar, and then you still step on the scale and the scale shows you that the weight has still increased. How frustrating is this.

I was personally frustrated about it multiple times and you often do not know what the right answer is when you get into a similar situation. In many cases the only seemingly reasonable answer is "**this**

damn thing simply does not work". it is just a

black magic, somehow this dietician lied to me so

let me just go and get my great dinner and let me

just forget about this as a nightmare because it

does not work anyway.

So, on the one hand this is true. Right, you need to

apply LOTS of effort in the course of several weeks

or a month. And it can be a very long process so it

feels like forever and the weight does not move.

And then there is no reward, right? So what do you

do about it how do you survive this and how do you

keep going?

In my case I had lots of frustrations and I also many

times simply broke those good habits and fell back

into the bad old habits just to realize later: no this

was not a good response. Let me go back but in

this case you have to go back after again gaining

several more pounds and just getting a journey a lot longer than you wanted it to be.

So what I learned in my case, which is the best thing about weight management that we previously discussed.

This best thing is energy in and energy out. As soon as you deeply internalize it, as soon as you deeply believe in it and you learn to ignore what numbers on the scale show you, you put yourself on a track to success. Guaranteed, taking no chances.

And assuming you persist, persist, persist and you wait, wait, wait - the numbers will eventually become more reasonable and the numbers you manage and deeply care about will get in touch with reality. This is the way for you to get through those hard times and this is the way how you can deal with this worst thing about weight

management.

And honestly I think it is a good life lesson as well.

Because in life there is no short-term metric you

can target and just see if you are doing well or not

you can look at the money in your bank account

genuinely if it goes up it is probably good.

But is it a good success metric in life? Probably not,

right, because if you simply target number of dollars

in your bank account at any given time, you will

miss on valuable opportunities and fail at solving

the real problem. You will miss on some good

education opportunities. You will not go spend

quality time with your friends or not entertain in

general. You will not invest in opportunities which

will long term both increase your balance in the

bank account and make other aspects of your life better.

So the weight management is probably another area which can make you more skilled managing something which on the one hand does exist, but on the other hand is not always the right thing to manage at the moment. The number is always there and if you step on the scale you know it.

But this number does not always move according to again what laws of physics and common sense would predict. If you starve yourself several days if you do not get enough energy you would expect your weight to go down simply because this energy burns the mass of your body.

But the problem with variation of the water weight in your body and some other unpredictability is that predictability of results in weight management effort could be a lot better.

So there needs to be some framework in your mind which should believe in which we deeply believe in and which just makes you persist right. it is just like faith but it is a different kind of faith in my case is just again faith in the fact that energy and preservation law is profound law. If your energy in is lower than the energy out for a long period of time then the results will follow and you just need to wait for a long enough period of time. And also the key to waiting this long period of time is to figuring out again what is sustainable. That's why I'm not a huge fan of diets and diets they may work to get more successful with weight management.

However long-term it is very hard to make

sustainable change to your life which you do not enjoy right.

So I suggest you still experiment and ideally find the ways that you <u>enjoy or at least can deal with over the long period of time,</u> and that can help you sustain. Sustain through this long, long period of time that is required to get your work for weight management efforts bring fruit.

This was the part about the worst thing about weight management. The worst thing about weight management is its unpredictability in a short term. Simply because there is lots of variations which you cannot deal with in predictable ways, the water weight is one of them. The water weight can make it look as if your weight management effort does not work and as if it is not worth it.

My best and only advice to you is believe in more

profound laws such as energy conservation, or

"energy in, energy out" as I referred to it earlier.

The law of conservation of energy is a great law to

believe in. Understand what your 'energy in' is,

what your 'energy out' is and over the what period

of time you should be losing what amount of

weight. Then just stick to the plan. Eventually you

will be rewarded. I promise.

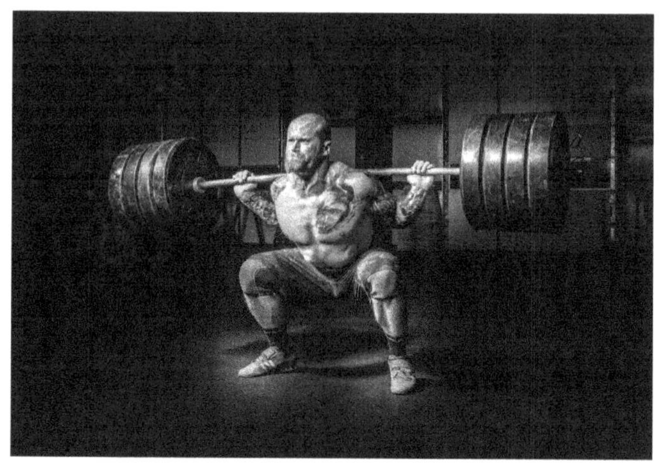

Why exercise is NOT a

weight management tool

Now let us talk about exercise.

I wanted to put my thoughts on this topic together

for quite a long time. It is a very important part of

this book and probably the important message that

I want to communicate and express my opinion about. It is also probably one of the most important points, which I hope will make this book different from other ones about managing your weight. I hope it will save you plenty of time and effort, set correct realistic expectations upfront and also will get you a better quality of life without broken promises to yourself and others.

Short summary is: **I do not believe exercise is a good weight management tool**. It is a bold statement, which goes directly against most common advice that people get when they want to lose weight - start exercising. So let me clarify this point it and explain what I mean by this.

Exercise is still great and totally worth it anyway

First, let me make it totally clear upfront that I deeply believe exercise is a great thing to do. It makes your life better. Exercise gets your muscles working, it gets your endorphins levels up, so you feel great after it. I know if first hand as I was a competitive swimmer a while ago and spent countless hours doing laps in the pool, and still trying to keep some of these good habits. Exercise is great in general, you should be doing it, and chances are you should be doing more of it. With regular exercise your life is going to improve quite noticeably; you are going to enjoy life a lot more with exercise and have more energy to do what you love and what matters.

However, while exercise is great for you in general and has lots of advantages, many people start exercising for the wrong reason, which is the main problem and the topic for this chapter. When these people come to a realize they need to lose weight, they believe exercise is the way to go to manage their weight.

And the fitness industry and a number of others amplify this message to reinforce this belief and make a living of it. All at your expense.

The fitness industry makes you commit to certain fitness goals over the course of a year. There is lots of pressure for you to exercise. And as a result first several weeks of the year there is no way to find a parking spot or empty machine in most gyms.

Then after two or three weeks or a month the New Year's resolution crowd is basically gone. With broken expectations, broken promises and goals not accomplished. There is nothing good about it. That's not cool and my goal is to simply explain to you that I do not believe exercise is a great weight management tool so you don't try it first.

If you are trying to manage your weight maybe you should start with exploring other tools that actually do work. And then when you are ready you can start using exercise for what it is worth as a fitness and life quality tool good for your well-being.

So why is exercise not a good weight management tool? As a product manager, I always think about the root cause of the problem that I'm dealing with. it is really important to solve the problem successfully instead of alleviating the symptom for a while and getting back to solving an amplified problem a bit later. You really need to understand what the root cause is and how this this root cause

can be addressed, what's the best way to fix it.

The root cause of weight gain

Let us talk about weight management and weight gain. What is the root cause of weight gain? Could it possibly be lack of exercise? Maybe, but if you say Yes, I would disagree. I could partially agree that yes, if you exercised more in the beginning then probably you would not be as much overweight as you are.

But the root cause for the weight gain is the excess energy intake as compared to energy expense. That's the only wait our body can accumulate weight, not counting temporary fluctuations in water weight. In most cases this means you simply eat too much. So you need to reduce your food intake for weight gain to slow down or for weight gain to stop or for weight loss to begin.

If you have inconsistent and unsustainable food consumption habits and you start to fix this energy gap by exercising more, I am more than sure you will be one of those people that eventually stop going to the gym and get disappointed in themselves. And even get maybe disappointed in your ability to stick to the promise, which was first of all not a good promise to give.

So what would be a better way for us to address the problem of weight management instead of going to the gym? If you look into the root cause, you understand that your weight is determined mostly by how much you eat how much energy you spend during the day. And if you do not spend enough, maybe you need to take an extra walk. Or maybe you need to get less food in your fridge.

There are certain small hacks like the less food you

have in your fridge the more likely you are to go somewhere and buy what you need. And when you go somewhere, it introduces friction in the system. Next time you want to eat something you will think twice: well I need to go buy it and maybe I do not want it badly enough so let me maybe not eat it now and I'm gonna go buy it later. And often we mistake thirst for hunger so you may drink some water and see if the hunger goes away.

So, keeping less food to the fridge is one small hack that could be used to manage your weight.

Wrong perception of energy amount your exercise burns

There are several other problems with exercise you need to be aware of.

First problem is that most people do not adequately understand the amount of energy they burn in the gym. Because of the way human brain works, I guess you may have experienced it multiple times as I did.

You exercise really hard, you sweat, you are exhausted so you believe that you've spent an insane amount of energy. And it just feels like you have done so much work. So you feel like you can definitely eat something you can reward yourself with some food. And even if you do not feel so, you are still really hungry anyway.

And the way it works, after exercising you will simply start eating way more than you burn in the gym. If you burned, say, 500 calories or so in the gym which is pretty meaningful exercise like half an hour run, the only reward you can afford for it is basically not even a whole burger, because a burger get you about a thousand calories.

So it is very likely that if you increase your food consumption that your energy balance will get even further out of whack. Consider an example where your energy input goes 1,000 calories higher (a burger or a burrito) and your energy expenditure is 500 calories higher. Net gain is another 500 calories per day, so over the course of the week you can gain another pound instead of losing a pound. This is insanely confusing and frustrating, so I hope you never deal with this.

Sustainable food consumption habits

And then finally imagine that you are not drawn to all those biases we discussed before and imagine you are a very rational person. And you calculate everything you eat, you do not indulge, and you are super strict with food so you are able to actually reduce the weight by adding exercise into your routines.

As many of my friends actually do it and they're pretty happy about it. So they asked me do you still believe that in this case it is still a bad tool for weight management. And yes I still believe so. I still believe exercise is a pretty bad weight management tool and the reason for this is as follows. Even if you are able to control your food intake so that your weight goes down during the course of your exercise period it is safe to assume you are not going to stick to this. Unless you really love exercising but if you really loved exercise you would probably not go overweight to start with.

So I guess something made you start doing this other than you enjoying it genuinely. And when you exercise and you eat in a way that weight goes down, it is **still not sustainable eating pattern** anyway because it includes the exercise energy expenditure in it.

So the first day that you stop exercising your food habits have already been shaped and you will continue eating roughly the same amount of same foods as if you exercised. And if you think about it, when your food habits have not adjusted after you stopped exercising and your previous energy deficit was simply there because of the exercise, there is a problem.

You have not done the most important thing: you have not adjusted your food intake and you have not adjusted your food habits. You will get back into the same positive balance of Energy IN vs. Energy OUT and your weight will keep creeping up. And the success of this whole initiative is not going to happen.

That's why I deeply believe exercise is NOT a good weight management tool. It is a great life quality tool, it is a great fitness tool, so it is a great thing to do. I strongly encourage you to exercise: figure out what you love, figure out what you enjoy and just do it as much as you enjoy but be honest. Do not think of exercise as a weight management tool, try to figure out the food consumption habits first, to figure out routines which will make you maintain your weight.

As soon as you figure out those food habits that can be an amazing step forward. This is something not many people actually ever figure out in their lives. And then on top of this accomplishment you will be able to introduce extra exercise.

And maybe you will fine tune your food intake a little bit for this because the exercise but only do this AFTER you figured out the food intake habit's which allow you to maintain your weight or make it go down without exercise in place.

Do not start exercising assuming is a great weight management tool - it is not.

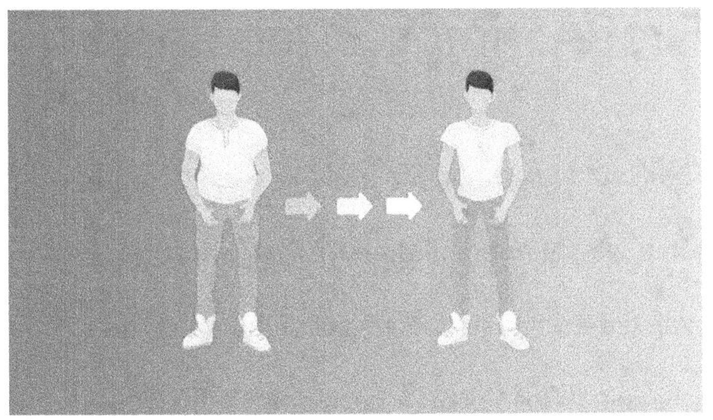

My personal experience losing weight

Now let me talk about my experience managing weight over the course of the last 5 years. Within these five years, I was able to lose more than 50 pounds twice. Within these five years, I was able to lose more than 50 pounds twice.

First Attempt: Brute Force

The first time I thought about the need to drop some weight happened about five years ago. That exercise was quite successful in the short term: I was able to lose quite a substantial amount of weight by making adjustment to food habits, ramping up exercise and generally making lifestyle more active, plus also added energy hacks such as sleeping without blanket that helped to burn hundreds incremental calories each day and speed up progress quite a bit.

But with short term success in a longer term that first attempt was not successful as all the weight came back after a short while. Looking back, the reason it happened was because because I did not think about weight management as a journey, but

rather as a one time heroic act and failed to form
new habits.

So everything I'm sharing with you in this book I
was not able to understand back then. I
characterized this first weight management or
weight loss attempt it was basically a Brute Force.
I realized that my body was getting out of shape
and out of control, so I had to do something about
it. At that time I discovered the "4-hour Body" book
by Tim Ferriss and many people were
recommending it and it promised some magic
transformation and deterministic path to feeling and
looking great, exactly what I was looking for.
And I just decided that I was doing to succeed
whatever it takes, or to simply power through the
difficulties which was a good fit with my character.

Five Rules from 4 Hour Body

5 rules from Tim Ferriss book that inspired my weight management effort 5 years ago

1. **First rule is to eliminate white carbs** or anything that can be white like rice or white flour. So replace those simple carbs into more complex carbs like brown rice instead of white.

2. **Second rule is to eat the same 3 meals over and over again**. Do not eat too many different things.

3. **Third rule was "Do not drink calories"** and this was a revelation to me. I was previously under impression that for instance juices were a pretty healthy food as they are made out of healthy fruits,

contain vitamins, etc. In my childhood I
drank a lot of juice but I never gained any
weight. So I always assumed juices are
great and other drinks are generally not so
bad for the body. So this was a revelation
for me when I realized there were so many
calories in those juices and juices are in
most cases just pure sugar and bring
nothing but harm to the body. So one by far
the most useful piece of advice from this
Timothy Ferris book for me was that fruit
juices are bad for health and generally
calories should not come from liquids. This
is the one rule I consider great and still
follow, while I do not follow many other
rules.

4. **Fourth rule is do not eat fruit.** I'm now
    pretty skeptical about it and will just say I
    understand their rationale that there is a lot
    sugar in the fruits, which leads to spike in
    blood sugar followed by spike in insulin,
    which is not good. t the time I did follow this
    advice, but now I made my choice in favor
    of keeping fruits in my diet, especially
    doubling down on berries.

5. **Fifth rule is Cheat Day**: take one day per
    week 'off' from following rules and go nuts.
    That's a tough one - I do not know how to
    feel about it, while Tim strongly
    recommends it to maintain sanity. I now
    believe you better build sustainable food
    consumption habits which do not require
    Cheat Day or any other rule to maintain

sanity. Because once a week is just not enough anyway to compensate for all all the effort restricting yourself six other days. I do not believe it is sustainable anyway. You will not be able to go through your whole life and limit your food intake to only reward yourself once a week. I think it is good for short-term exercise to gain confidence that you can both follow the healthy rules and control your body. Long term I do not think it is a good thing to do I as there are better ways.

Physics and Key Levers to Burn More Energy

Not super excited about being a slave to arbitrary rules, I tried to figure out other ways of weight management which allow to less constrain my food intake and make it less of a heroic effort.

So, I realized as a past physicist that there are several other levers to impact your energy balance not related to food intake.

Mechanics

Remembering about mechanics, moving mass over a distance burns energy. Most people manipulate energy balance through exercise: they run, swim, bike etc. Which I also did but the disadvantages of creating extra energy deficit via exercise is that to burn any meaningful amount of energy, you have to work out A LOT. Like running 1 hour for a close to 200 pound male would burn about a 1,000 calories, an energy you consume by eating a burger. And if you do not truly enjoy the exercise, you won't last long even if it helps you get to some short term results.

I actually did lots of exercise that time - biking, running, swimming - so I did not follow my own today's advice about exercise not being a weight management tool. I just went overboard and did everything to succeed fastest possible way.

Thermodynamics

But in addition to mechanics there is also thermodynamics. As I thought about it more creatively there is actually another easy natural way for you to burn more energy. For example, if you live in a cold climate you need to eat plenty of heavy food full of calories just to survive. Because people spend a lot of extra energy being outside in the frost that the body needs to maintain heat. So you spend a lot of energy to just maintain your body temperature, which makes sense remembering that body temperature is 36 degrees Celsius and the outside temperature on a cold day could be negative 25 or so, which is a 60 degrees delta. Checking web sources, we find that average adult inhales and exhales about 11,000 liters of air per day or 500 liters per hour or 8 liters per minute. So if you spend an hour in negative 25 frost outside, breathing in roughly 500 liters of air (and applying heat capacity of air 1.006 kJ/kgC, density of air at 1.225 kg/m^3 or 0.6 kg mass of air in 500 liters) we get to energy burn of 0.6 kg x 1.006 kJ/kgC x 60 degrees delta = **36 kJ** or in calories (Kilocalories) divided by 4,200 **roughly 9 calories**.

That does not sound like a lot but those calories do add up. And that gives you two powerful levers, both time and temperature, which is great.

My big learning from this was: what if this same principle can be used to increase energy expenditure when you sleep. If you keep lowering your room temperature when you sleep, you do not care what it is as long as you can still sleep the whole night. This is one tool that I realized that could be useful and I was just experimenting with a

thermostat temperature. Changing it in the way that

you can still sleep the whole night but so that you

can reduce this temperature. Assuming you sleep

for 8 hours, breathing in and out 4,000 liters of air =

4 kg of air weight, moving the room temperature

down by just 1 degree can help create an extra 1+

calorie energy deficit. Does not sound like a lot, but

it made me think further.

And the second thing about the thermodynamics I

also figured out that if you sleep without blanket or

with a thin blanket that help air circulate, you create

an extra energy deficit because of the difference in

skin temperature and the air temperature. This tool

is a little bit of an extreme so not everybody can do

it or at least not during most of the year. But if you

sleep without the blanket your body obviously burns

even more energy because it does not retain the air which is just warmed up under the blanket.

If there is no blanket then you consistently radiate the energy of the course of a night and it can be up to three hundred or so calories. Really, it can actually be a pretty substantial amount of energy which is quite a useful tool to balance your energy equation.

My logic at that time was if I have a choice to exercise an hour in the gym or to sleep without the blanket. Which one would I choose? And I'm pretty lazy person, so I preferred sleeping without a blanket and this was actually working like magic. I could see a weight going down very substantially over time without crazy constraints on food. I still believe sleeping without a blanket is a great way of burning more energy as long as you can sustain it.

My creative approach at that time gave several other ideas, some of which I did not even see anywhere online. For example, we know that heart consumes roughly 20% of all our resting energy to pump the blood. This amount of energy is higher when we stand than when we sit because of the gravity and the work that heart needs to do to move the mass of the blood up. So the idea was what if your bed is not ideally horizontal but a little bit sloped upwards - like 5 degrees. It does seem like that results in higher energy expense similar to additional exercise in nature, and not clear how it would impact the sleep quality. I never tried this idea but excited to find new ones and discuss. And today I do not have to do this anymore as I believe I figured out even better ways to keep the energy balance.

If you really need to lose weight, if you need to do it faster, you can think of using this tool sleeping without a blanket is a good thing to consider.

I did everything at once: changed my food intake,ramped up exercise and generally activity levels during the day, I started sleeping without the blanket and did whatever it takes to burn more energy while also consuming less. That effort was a success and it happened so fast that it gave me a sense of being super powerful in terms of controlling my body. Up to the level that I believed I could do it anytime.

And when I changed the job that came with extra stress and reduced the level of discipline with food consumption, the weight quickly came back up.

And then second journey of trying to put weight back down was a pretty tough challenge. So, the main thing I learned from that period of working

hard getting weight down and then within three to

six months getting it all back was that there must be

a better more sustainable way. And I had to find it.

Sustainable Habits

Now my approach to health and weight management can be summarized with a word **sustainability**. You need to figure out what works for you, you need to forget about immediate results and instant gratification, and just need to understand and accept this is going to be a lifetime journey. It's never going to end.

Think of it for example just like about your career. You need to manage your career all the time, actively, success is not a result of one month brute force effort. Weight management is a long term exercise, it is a long journey and as you go with this journey you figure out what works for you and what does not.

So, my biggest learning which I'm sharing here is about fasting and generally constraining energy intake over a certain period of time, instead of constraining the types of foods or number of times you eat.

There are different kinds of fasting. Fasting stands generally for not eating anything for a period of say one or two days. But there is also a concept of intermittent fasting where you keep eating the same amount of energy during the course of the day. You just increase the interval of time that you spend without eating any food. For instance intermittent fasting with sixteen-hour window would mean that you can eat within 8 hour time window and for sixteen hours you do not eat anything. Your total calorie intake can stay the same.

What I learned that for me intermittent fasting is a lot more sustainable to not constrain my food intake choices. It only takes learning to deal with hunger for a limited period of time. As long as you can deal with hunger psychologically and you can just go through this period of time you can then enjoy your normal food and you can enjoy your normal life. You do not have to make crazy adjustments, do not need to sleep without a blanket or to forget about rice if you like rice.

So to me this was a reasonable trade-off. Even if it is a choice to learn how to fast versus the choice of giving up my favorite foods I would rather learn how to fast and I got increasingly better psychologically handling periods without food.

And then the final tool which is even more extreme I do not recommend it to you until you at least get more comfortable with normal fasting and get approval from your doctor. There is a tool called dry fasting which restricts consumption not of just food but also water. And the reasoning behind dry fasting is this puts your body into such a stress mode that it burns a lot more energy a lot faster. And it also burns fat in this case to get water, not just to release energy. If you only burned fat for energy, you would be burning a pound of fat to get 3,500 calories of energy. If you do not eat anything for two days you would expect a pound of fat loss. In case of dry fast your body burns fat much faster because it also uses it as the water storage. I do not have precise numbers but in one three day dry fast it is reasonable to expect about a 10 pound total weight loss, which would both include water weight and fat weight. Again, this is not just fat -

you are going to gain much of it back but the immediate results in terms of how you look and feel will be absolutely fantastic.

Summary

This was my personal experience losing weight. First time via a Brute Force approach, combining food adjustments, lots of exercise and energy body hacks. I learned lots of new things by trying lots of different methods combined and it got me to desired results super-fast. But that first time I did not follow sustainable set of rules, so as a result I gained everything back and even more.
And then the second time I did a lot better job figuring out what works best for me, and what trade offs are the best. So it took a lot longer time but I believe I figured out a sustainable way without

going into any kind of extremes. I believe this experimentation makes you way more powerful in terms of weight management and generally understanding which levers you have to get to results. Learning new tools allows living a better healthier life while still keeping your weight under control.